About the NCCN Guidelines for Patients®

NCCN National Comprehensive Cancer Network®

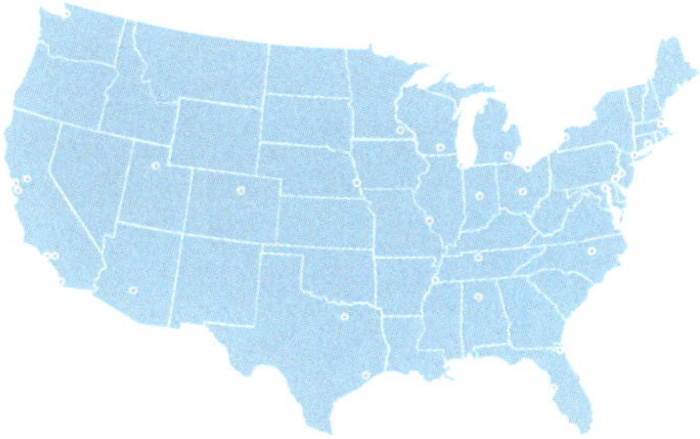

Did you know that top cancer centers across the United States work together to improve cancer care? This alliance of leading cancer centers is called the National Comprehensive Cancer Network® (NCCN®).

Cancer care is always changing. NCCN develops evidence-based cancer care recommendations used by health care providers worldwide. These frequently updated recommendations are the NCCN Clinical Practice Guidelines in Oncology (NCCN Guidelines®). The NCCN Guidelines for Patients plainly explain these expert recommendations for people with cancer and caregivers.

These NCCN Guidelines for Patients are based on the NCCN Clinical Practice Guidelines in Oncology (NCCN Guidelines®) for Head and Neck Cancers Version 2.2024 – December 8, 2023.

View the NCCN Guidelines for Patients free online
NCCN.org/patientguidelines

Find an NCCN Cancer Center near you
NCCN.org/cancercenters

Connect with us

Supporters

NCCN Guidelines for Patients are supported by funding from the NCCN Foundation®

NCCN independently adapts, updates, and hosts the NCCN Guidelines for Patients. Our corporate supporters do not participate in the development of the NCCN Guidelines for Patients and are not responsible for the content and recommendations contained therein.

To make a gift or learn more, visit online or email

NCCNFoundation.org/donate

PatientGuidelines@NCCN.org

Contents

NCCN Foundation seeks to support the millions of patients and their families affected by a cancer diagnosis by funding and distributing NCCN Guidelines for Patients. NCCN Foundation is also committed to advancing cancer treatment by funding the nation's promising doctors at the center of innovation in cancer research. For more details and the full library of patient and caregiver resources, visit NCCN.org/patients.

National Comprehensive Cancer Network (NCCN) and NCCN Foundation
3025 Chemical Road, Suite 100, Plymouth Meeting, PA 19462 USA

1
NPC basics

Nasopharyngeal carcinoma (NPC) is a type of cancer that affects the nasopharynx. The nasopharynx connects the back of the nose (nasal cavity) to the back of the mouth (pharynx).

The pharynx

The pharynx is part of the throat and found inside the neck. It is a hollow, muscular tube that starts behind the nose (nasal cavity) and opens into the voice box (larynx) and esophagus (the tube that goes to the stomach).

The pharynx (said fair-inks) has 3 parts:

- Nasopharynx
- Oropharynx
- Hypopharynx

Cancer can be found in any part of the pharynx. This book will focus on cancer of the nasopharynx, also called nasopharyngeal carcinoma (NPC). The nasopharynx is a small, tube-shaped structure above the soft part of the back of the mouth (soft palate) that connects the nasal cavity to the oropharynx. The nasal cavity is the space inside the nose. It lies above the bone that forms the roof of the mouth (hard palate) and curves down at the back to join the throat. The oropharynx includes the back of the roof of the mouth (soft palate), the tonsils, the side and back walls of the throat, and the base of the tongue found in the throat.

The pharynx

The pharynx is a hollow, muscular tube inside the neck that starts behind the nose and opens into the larynx and esophagus. The pharynx has 3 parts: the nasopharynx, oropharynx, and hypopharynx.

Anatomy of the Pharynx

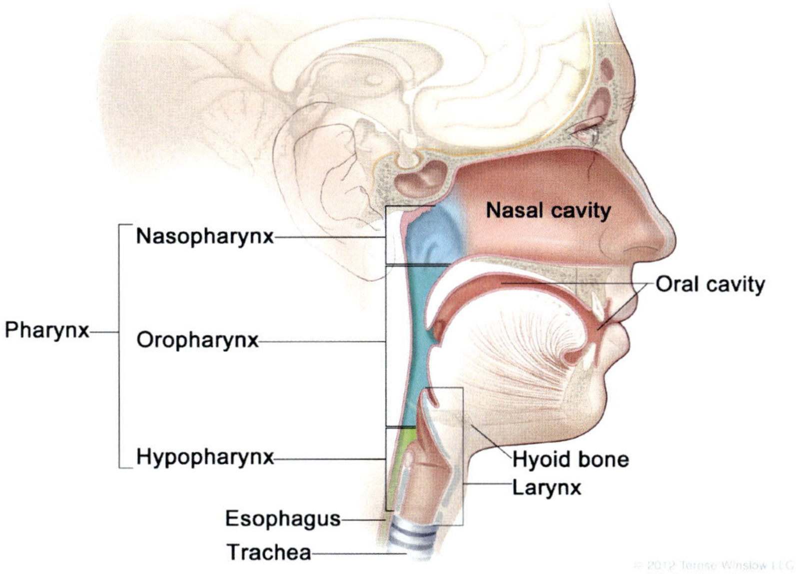

Head and neck cancer

Head and neck cancers are a group of cancers that arise in the head or neck area of the body. Cancer is named and treated based on the tumor location or where the cancer started.

Cancer can occur in the

- Mouth (oral cavity),
- Middle part of the throat near the mouth (oropharynx),
- Space behind the nose (nasal cavity and paranasal sinuses),
- Upper part of the throat near the nasal cavity (nasopharynx),
- Voice box (larynx), or
- Lower part of the throat near the larynx (hypopharynx).

More information on mouth cancer and throat (oropharyngeal) cancer can be found at NCCN.org/patientguidelines and on the NCCN Patient Guides for Cancer app.

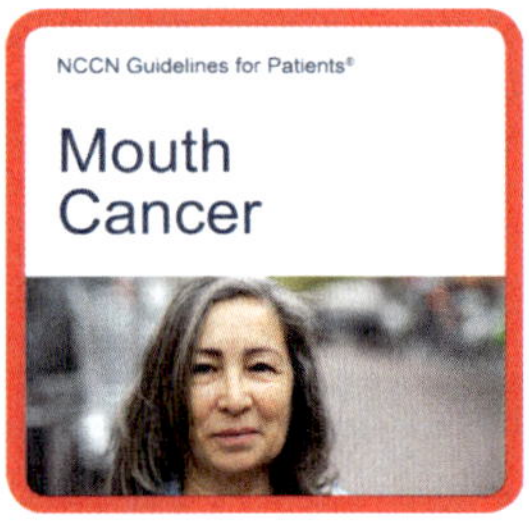

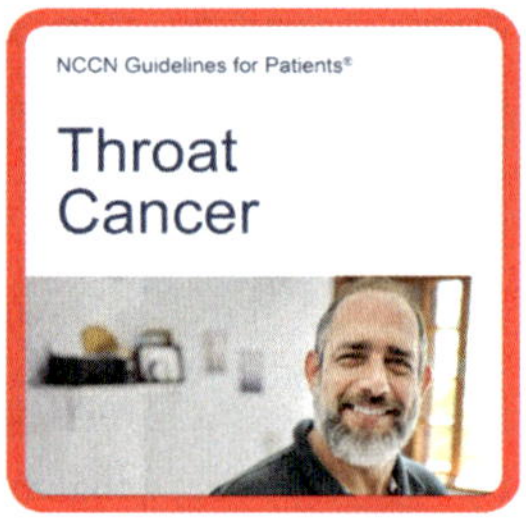

It is strongly recommended, when possible, for those with head and neck cancers to be treated at a high-volume center or hospital that has experience in their type of cancer.

Nasopharyngeal cancer

Nasopharyngeal cancer (NPC) is a rare cancer that most often occurs in people from parts of Asia, Native America, and North Africa. Most NPCs start in the squamous cells that form the surface lining of the nasopharynx. Normally, these are thin, flat cells and are similar to the top layer of skin and surface lining of some other parts of the body such as the lungs and esophagus. Squamous cell carcinoma (SCC) is the most common type of nasopharyngeal cancer and is the focus of this book.

Cancer cells form a tumor called a primary tumor within the area of the nasopharynx, the part of the throat connecting the back of the nose (nasal cavity) to the back of the mouth (the pharynx). A tumor can grow into nearby tissue. Cancer cells often spread to lymph nodes in the neck, and less frequently to the lungs.

It's often difficult to recognize nasopharyngeal cancer because the symptoms are similar to other less serious conditions. Also, many people with nasopharyngeal cancer don't have any symptoms until the cancer reaches an advanced stage.

Nasopharyngeal cancer shouldn't be confused with other types of cancer that also affect the throat, such as laryngeal cancer and esophageal cancer. More information on esophageal cancer can be found at NCCN.org/patientguidelines and on the NCCN Patient Guides for Cancer app.

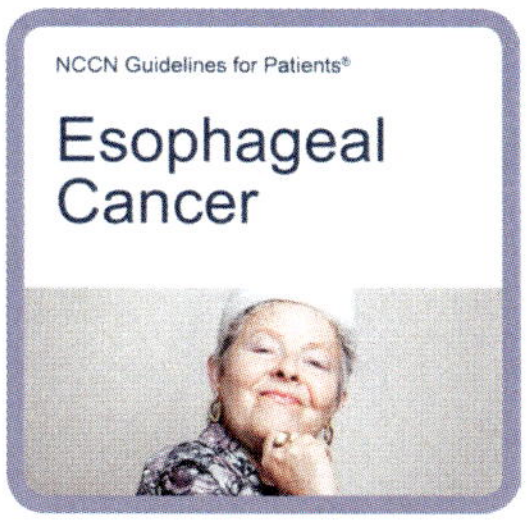

Key points

- Nasopharyngeal carcinoma (NPC) is a type of cancer that affects the nasopharynx.
- The nasopharynx connects the back of the nose (nasal cavity) to the back of the mouth (pharynx).
- Head and neck cancers are a group of cancers that arise in the head or neck area of the body.
- Cancer treatment is based on the tumor location.
- Squamous cell carcinoma (SCC) is the most common type of nasopharyngeal cancer. It forms in the thin, flat cells of the mucus membranes of the nasopharynx. SCC is the focus of this book.

2
Testing for NPC

Treatment planning starts with testing. This chapter presents an overview of the tests you might receive and what to expect.

Test results

Results from medical history, physical examination, imaging studies, and biopsy will be used to determine your treatment plan. Treatment will be based on these findings. It is important you understand what these tests mean. Ask questions and keep copies of your test results. Online patient portals are a great way to access your test results. Discuss your results with your health care provider (HCP).

Keep these things in mind:

- Find out where your insurance allows you to be treated. Seek out a comprehensive cancer center with doctors who are experts in evaluating and treating nasopharyngeal carcinoma (NPC). You'll want to do this step early on.
- Choose a friend, family member, or peer who can drive you to appointments, provide meals, or offer emotional support during diagnosis and treatment.
- Bring someone with you to doctor visits, if possible.
- Write down questions and take notes during appointments. Don't be afraid to ask your care team questions. Get to know your care team and help them get to know you.
- Get copies of blood tests, imaging results, and reports about the specific type of cancer you have.
- Organize your papers. Create files for insurance forms, medical records, and test results. You can do the same on your computer.
- Keep a list of contact information for everyone on your care team. Add it to your phone. Hang the list on your refrigerator or keep it in a place where someone can access it in an emergency. Keep your primary care physician (PCP) informed of changes to this list. You are encouraged to keep your PCP in the loop. They are great partners in your care.
- In your contact list, include information on the exact type of cancer you have, as well as any treatments you've received and the date each treatment started.

For possible tests, **see Guide 1.**

General health tests

Some general health tests are described next. You will not have all of these tests.

Medical history

A medical history is a record of all health issues and treatments you have had in your life. Be prepared to list any illness or injury and when it happened. Bring a list of old and new medicines and any over-the-counter (OTC) medicines, herbals, or supplements you take. Some supplements interact with and affect medicines that your care team may prescribe. Tell your care team about any symptoms you have. A medical history, sometimes called a health history, will help determine which treatment is best for you.

Guide 1
Tests for treatment planning

Medical history, tobacco and alcohol use history, and physical exam, including complete head and neck exam. Mirror exam if needed. Screen for depression.
Nasopharyngeal fiberoptic exam
Biopsy of tumor or neck
MRI with contrast of collarbone to skull base. CT of skull base and neck may also be done.
Imaging for distant metastases with FDG-PET/CT and/or chest CT with contrast
As needed: • Epstein-Barr virus (EBV) DNA testing • Dental exam • Nutrition, speech, and swallowing evaluation, and hearing test (audiogram) • Eye and endocrine evaluation • Help to quit smoking • Fertility counseling

Family history

NPC most often occurs in those from parts of Asia, Native America, and North Africa. Head and neck cancers are not inherited from your biological parents. However, some cancers and other diseases can run in families. Your care team will ask about the health history of family members who are blood relatives. This information is called a family history. Ask family members on both sides of your family about their health issues like heart disease, cancer, and diabetes, and at what age they were diagnosed. It's important to know the specific type of cancer or where the cancer started, if it is in multiple locations, and if they had genetic testing.

Tobacco and alcohol use history

Tobacco and alcohol use are known risk factors for developing head and neck cancer and can limit how well treatment works. Their use can affect survival. You will be asked about your tobacco and alcohol use history and asked to avoid tobacco and limit alcohol use during treatment. Speak to your care team if you have any questions or concerns.

Physical exam

During a physical exam, your health care provider may:

- Check your temperature, blood pressure, pulse, and breathing rate
- Check your height and weight
- Listen to your lungs and heart
- Look in your eyes, ears, nose, and throat
- Feel and apply pressure to parts of your body to see if organs are of normal size, are soft or hard, or cause pain when touched.
- Feel for enlarged lymph nodes in your neck, underarm, and groin.

Complete head and neck exam

A physical exam will include the head and neck. Since the oropharynx is found inside the throat, some parts are not easy to see when you open your mouth. A health care provider might use a special mirror or fiberoptic scope to look at these areas.

Dental exam

It is important to tell your dentist about your head and neck cancer and to have regular dental cleanings and checkups. Head and neck cancer and its treatment can affect the health of your jaw, teeth, and gums. If you need any dental work or procedures, they might be recommended before starting certain treatments.

Distress screening

It is normal to have strong feelings about being diagnosed with cancer, and your feelings can change from day to day and week to week. Talk to your care team and those whom you feel most comfortable about how you are feeling. There are services and people who can help you. Support and counseling are available. Many treatment teams include mind and body therapists who can help.

Dealing with a cancer diagnosis can be stressful and may cause further distress. Distress is an unpleasant experience of a mental, physical, social, or spiritual nature. It can affect how you feel, think, and act. Distress might include feelings of sadness, fear, helplessness, worry, anger, and guilt. You may also experience depression, anxiety, and sleep issues. Your treatment team will screen your level of distress. This is part of your cancer care.

Eye exam

Sometimes, nasopharyngeal cancer can affect the eyes. An eye exam might be recommended before starting treatment.

Endocrine tests

Radiation therapy to the head and neck can affect endocrine (hormone) glands found in the head and neck, such as thyroid and pituitary glands. Therefore, blood tests to look at thyroid endocrine levels might be done before and/or after treatment.

Hearing test

A hearing test shows if there is any hearing loss, and if so, the type of hearing loss, how severe it is, and what might have caused it. An audiogram is a graph showing the results of a pure-tone hearing test. Tumors in the head and neck can affect hearing. Treatment of head and neck tumors can also affect hearing.

Nutrition assessment

You might meet with a nutrition expert before starting treatment. A nutritionist or dietician can suggest the best foods and fluids for you. It is important that you receive adequate and sustained nutrition before you start treatment.

Speech and swallowing assessment

You might visit with a speech or swallowing therapist who will test your ability to swallow and speak before and after treatment.

Performance status

Performance status (PS) is a person's general level of fitness and ability to perform daily self-care tasks. It is one factor taken into consideration when choosing a treatment plan. Your preferences about treatment are always important.

Fertility (all genders)

Treatment such as chemotherapy can affect your fertility, the ability to have children. If you think you want children in the future, ask your care team how cancer and cancer treatment might change your fertility. To preserve your fertility, you may need to take action before starting cancer treatment. Those who want to have children in the future should be referred to a fertility specialist to discuss the options before starting treatment.

Fertility preservation is all about keeping your options open, whether you know you want to have children later in life or aren't really sure at the moment. Fertility and reproductive specialists can help you sort through what may be best for your situation.

More information on fertility preservation in adolescents and young adults is available at NCCN.org/patientguidelines and on the NCCN Patient Guides for Cancer app.

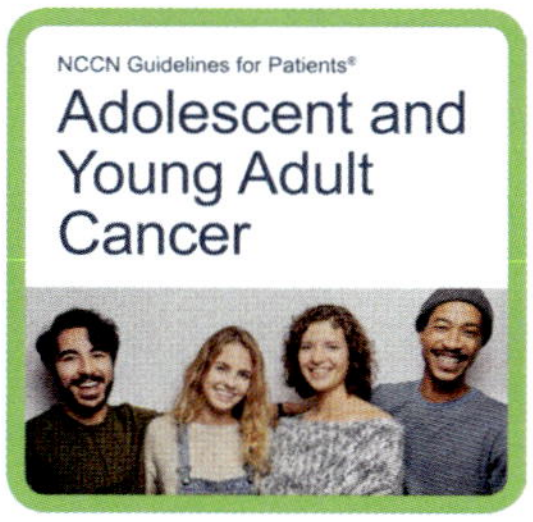

Changes in fertility

Treatment might cause your fertility to be temporarily or permanently impaired or interrupted. This loss of fertility is related to your age at time of diagnosis, treatment type(s), treatment dose, and treatment length. Talk to your care team about your concerns and if you are planning a pregnancy.

Preventing pregnancy during treatment

Preventing pregnancy during treatment is important. Cancer and cancer treatment can affect the ovaries and damage sperm. Hormonal birth control may or may not be recommended, so ask your doctor about options such as intrauterine devices (IUDs) and barrier methods. Types of barrier methods include condoms, diaphragms, cervical caps, and the contraceptive sponge.

Those with ovaries

Those who can become pregnant will have a pregnancy test before starting treatment. Cancer treatment can hurt the developing baby if you are or become pregnant during treatment. Therefore, birth control to prevent pregnancy during and after treatment is recommended. If you are pregnant or breastfeeding at the time of your cancer diagnosis, certain treatments will need to be avoided.

Menstruation, menses, menstrual flow, or your "period" may stop during treatment, but often returns within 2 years after treatment in those 35 years of age and under. It is still possible to become pregnant even though you might not have a period. Therefore, birth control is recommended during and after treatment. Consult your doctor for the best time to plan a pregnancy.

Imaging tests

Imaging tests take pictures of the inside of your body. Imaging tests show the primary tumor, or where the cancer started, and look for cancer in other parts of the body. A radiologist, an expert in interpreting imaging tests, will write a report and send this report to your health care provider (HCP). It is likely that the report will be sent directly to you through your patient portal or patient access system. You should discuss these results with your HCP. You will not have all of the following tests.

Contrast material

Contrast material is used to improve the pictures of the inside of the body. Contrast materials are not dyes, but substances that help enhance and improve the images of several organs and structures in the body. It is used to make the pictures clearer. The contrast is not permanent and will leave your body in your urine immediately after the test. The types of contrast vary and are different for CT and MRI.

Tell your care team if you have had allergic reactions to contrast in the past. This is important. You might be given medicines to avoid the effects of those allergies. Contrast might not be used if you have a serious allergy or if your kidneys aren't working well.

If you smoke or vape, seek help to quit

A history of smoking or vaping nicotine increases your chances of developing head and neck, lung, and other cancers. Smoking and vaping can limit how well cancer treatment works and prevent wound healing. They also greatly increase your chances of having side effects during and after surgery. Cannabis use might also affect the amount of anesthesia used during surgery.

Nicotine is the chemical in tobacco that makes you want to keep smoking and vaping. Nicotine withdrawal is challenging for most people who smoke or vape. The stress of having cancer may make it even harder to quit. If you smoke or vape, ask your care team about counseling and medicines to help you quit. In head and neck cancers, stopping smoking or vaping is essential to maximize the chance for cure and minimize side effects.

For online support, try these websites:

- SmokeFree.gov
- BeTobaccoFree.gov
- CDC.gov/tobacco

CT scan

A computed tomography (CT or CAT) scan uses x-rays and computer technology to take pictures of the inside of the body. It takes many x-rays of the same body part from different angles. All the images are combined to make one detailed picture. A CT scan of your head, neck, and chest may be one of the tests to look for cancer. In most cases, contrast will be used.

MRI scan

A magnetic resonance imaging (MRI) scan uses radio waves and powerful magnets to take pictures of the inside of the body. It does not use x-rays. Because of the very strong magnets used in the MRI machine, tell the technologist if you have any metal in your body. During the test, you will likely be asked to hold your breath for 10 to 20 seconds as the technician collects the images. Contrast is often used.

A closed MRI has a capsule-like design where the magnet surrounds you. An open MRI has a magnetic top and bottom, which allows for an opening on each end. Closed MRIs are more common than open MRIs, so if you have claustrophobia (a dread or fear of enclosed spaces), be sure to talk to your care team about it.

PET scan

A positron emission tomography (PET) scan uses a radioactive drug called a tracer. A tracer is a substance injected into a vein to see where cancer cells are in the body and if they are using sugar produced by your body to grow. Cancer cells show up as bright spots on PET scans. However, not all tumors will appear on a PET scan. Also, not all bright spots are cancer. It is normal for the brain, heart, kidneys, and bladder to be bright on PET. Inflammation or infection can also show up as a bright spot. When a PET scan is combined with CT, it is called a PET/CT scan.

FDG-PET/CT

An FDG-PET/CT uses a radiotracer called fluorodeoxyglucose (FDG). It is made of fluoride and a simple form of sugar called glucose. You cannot eat or drink for at least 4 hours before the scan. This scan is most helpful when other imaging results are unclear. It may help find cancer in lymph nodes and distant sites. If it clearly shows cancer in the bone, a bone scan and sodium fluoride PET/CT may not be needed. FDG-PET/CT can be done at the same time as a CT used for diagnosis.

Ultrasound

Ultrasound (US) uses high-energy sound waves to form pictures of the inside of the body. This is similar to the sonogram used for pregnancy. A wand-like probe (transducer) will be held and moved on your neck using gel. Ultrasound is painless and does not use x-rays, so it can be repeated as needed. Ultrasound is good at showing small areas of cancer that may be in lymph nodes. Sometimes, an ultrasound or CT is used to guide a fine-needle biopsy (FNB).

Panoramic dental x-ray

A panoramic dental x-ray or panoramic x-ray (Panorex) uses a very small dose of radiation to capture the entire mouth in one image, including the teeth, upper and lower jaw, and surrounding structures and tissues. It is commonly performed by dentists and oral surgeons in everyday practice and may be used to plan treatment for dentures, braces, extractions, and implants.

Biopsy

A biopsy removes a sample of tissue or fluid. Samples removed during a biopsy or surgery will be sent to a pathologist, an expert in examining cells using a microscope (called cytology) to confirm the presence of cancer. The pathologist will determine the cancer subtype called tumor histology.

A fine-needle aspiration (FNA), fine-needle biopsy (FNB), and core needle biopsy (CNB) use needles of different sizes to remove a sample of tumor or lymph node. An ultrasound or CT scan might be used to guide a lymph node biopsy.

Biopsy of metastasis

Metastasis is the spread of cancer to an area of the body such as lymph nodes or lung. A biopsy of the metastasis may be needed to confirm the presence of cancer. If there is more than one metastasis, each site may be biopsied. The type of biopsy used depends on the location of the suspected metastases and other factors.

Biomarker testing

Biomarker tumor testing includes tests of genes or their products (proteins). It identifies the presence or absence of mutations and certain proteins that might suggest treatment. This information is used to choose the best treatment for you. It is sometimes called molecular testing or tumor profiling, tumor sequencing, gene expression profiling, or genomic testing.

Inside our cells are deoxyribonucleic acid (DNA) molecules. These molecules are tightly packaged into what is called a chromosome. Chromosomes contain most of the genetic information in a cell. Normal human cells contain 23 pairs of chromosomes for a total of 46 chromosomes. Each chromosome contains thousands of genes. Genes are coded instructions for the proteins your cells make. Most genes contain information about a specific protein. A mutation is when something goes wrong in the genetic code.

Epstein-Barr virus

Epstein-Barr virus (EBV) is a common virus that causes infectious mononucleosis. It remains dormant or inactive in most people. Cancer caused by EBV is called EBV-related cancer. Most nasopharyngeal cancers are EBV-related. A sample of your tumor and/or blood will be tested for EBV DNA before and after treatment.

MSI-H/dMMR mutation

Microsatellites are short, repeated strings of DNA. When errors or defects occur, they are fixed by mismatch repair (MMR) proteins. Some cancers have DNA mutations or changes that prevent these errors from being fixed. This is called microsatellite instability (MSI) or deficient mismatch repair (dMMR). When cancer cells have more than a normal number of microsatellites, it is called MSI-H (microsatellite instability-high). This is often due to dMMR genes.

PD-L1 testing

Programmed death ligand 1 (PD-L1) is an immune protein. If this protein is expressed on the surface of cancer cells, it can cause your immune cells to ignore the cancer and suppress the anti-tumor immune response. If your cancer expresses this protein, you might have treatment that combines chemotherapy and an immune checkpoint inhibitor therapy. This is designed to activate your immune system to better fight off the cancer cells.

Tumor HPV testing

Human papillomavirus (HPV) is a group of viruses that infect the cells on the surface of skin or on the moist surfaces or inner linings of some organs and body cavities. HPV infection usually clears on its own. However, HPV infections can cause abnormal tissue growth (warts) and sometimes cancer. Cancer caused by HPV is called HPV-related cancer. In cancers of the head and neck, throat cancer is most often related to HPV. However, HPV testing might be done in some cases for nasopharyngeal cancer.

More information on HPV can be found in NCCN Guidelines for Patients: Throat Cancer, available at NCCN.org/patientguidelines and on the NCCN Patient Guides for Cancer app.

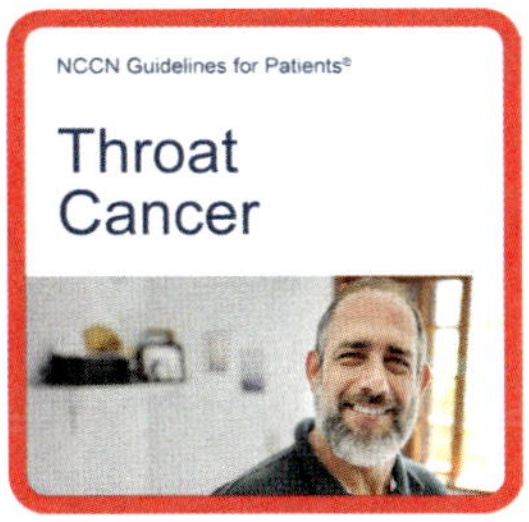

Tumor mutational burden

When there are 10 or more mutations per million base pairs of tumor DNA, it is called tumor mutational burden-high (TMB-H). Metastatic or unresectable TMB cancers are often treated using immunotherapy drugs that target the proteins called programmed cell death protein 1 (PD-1) or programmed death ligand 1 (PD-L1).

Tumor mutation testing

Tumor mutation testing or tumor genomic aberration testing uses a sample of your tumor or blood to see if the cancer cells have any specific DNA mutations. This is a different type of DNA testing than the genetic testing for mutations you may have inherited from your biological parents. In tumor mutation testing, only the tumor is tested and not the rest of your body. Some mutations can be targeted with specific therapies.

Key points

- Results from imaging studies and a biopsy will determine your treatment plan. Often, information is collected over time, even as treatment begins. Online portals are a great way to access your test results. Please discuss your results with your health care provider.
- A medical history and physical exam inform your care team about your overall health. Your overall health may guide the best treatment for your cancer.
- Head and neck cancer and its treatment can affect the health of your jaw, teeth, and gums. Tell your dentist about your head and neck cancer and keep up with regular dental cleanings and checkups.
- Treatment can affect fertility. Talk to your care team about your concerns and if you are planning a pregnancy.
- Imaging tests take pictures of the inside of your body.
- A biopsy removes a sample of tissue or fluid for testing.
- A sample of your tumor or blood may be tested to look for specific DNA (deoxyribonucleic acid) mutations, protein levels, or other molecular features. Some mutations and proteins can be targeted with specific therapies.
- Cancer caused by the Epstein-Barr virus (EBV) is called EBV-related cancer. Most nasopharyngeal cancers are EBV-related.

3

Nasopharyngeal cancer staging

Cancer staging is used to reflect prognosis and to guide treatment decisions. It describes the size and location of the tumor and if cancer has spread to lymph nodes or other parts of the body. This chapter explains nasopharyngeal carcinoma (NPC) stages.

How NPC is staged

A cancer stage is a way to describe the extent of the cancer at the time you are first diagnosed. The American Joint Committee on Cancer (AJCC) created a staging system to determine how much cancer is in your body, where it is located, and what subtype you have. This is called staging. Cancer staging is not the same for all cancer types and locations.

Based on testing, your cancer will be assigned a stage. Staging helps to predict prognosis and is needed to make treatment decisions. A prognosis is the course your cancer will likely take. AJCC is just one type of staging system.

Information gathered during staging:

- **The extent (size) of the tumor (T):** How large is the cancer? Has it grown into nearby areas?
- **The spread to nearby lymph nodes (N):** Has the cancer spread to nearby lymph nodes? If so, how many? Where?
- **The spread (metastasis) to distant sites (M):** Has the cancer spread to distant organs such as the lungs or liver?
- **Biomarker testing:** Does the cancer have any genes or mutations that might suggest treatment?

Staging is based on a combination of information to reach a final numbered stage. Often, not all information is available at the initial evaluation. More information can be gathered as treatment begins. Doctors may explain your cancer stage in different ways than described next.

Staging includes:

- **Anatomic –** based on extent of cancer as defined by tumor size (T), lymph node status (N), and distant metastasis (M).
- **Prognostic –** includes anatomic TNM and often Epstein-Barr virus (EBV) levels in the blood. The prognostic stage also includes the assumption that you are treated with the standard-of-care approaches.

Prognostic stages are divided into clinical and pathologic. Cancer staging is often done twice, before and after surgery. Staging after surgery provides more specific and accurate details about the size of the cancer and lymph node status.

Clinical stage

Clinical stage (c) is the rating given before any treatment. It is based on a physical exam, biopsy, and imaging tests. An example might look like cN2 or cM1. In nasopharyngeal cancer, the clinical stage is based on imaging and biopsy results. These tests are done before any treatment as part of an initial diagnosis.

Pathologic stage

Pathologic stage (p) or surgical stage is determined by examining tissue removed during surgery. An example might be pN2. If you are given cancer drug therapy before surgery, then the stage might add a "y" and look like ypT3.

How cancer can spread

Nasopharyngeal cancer can spread to nearby lymph nodes, and areas such as the nasal cavity, oropharynx, hypopharynx, base of the skull, jaw, and roof of the mouth.

Anatomy of the Pharynx

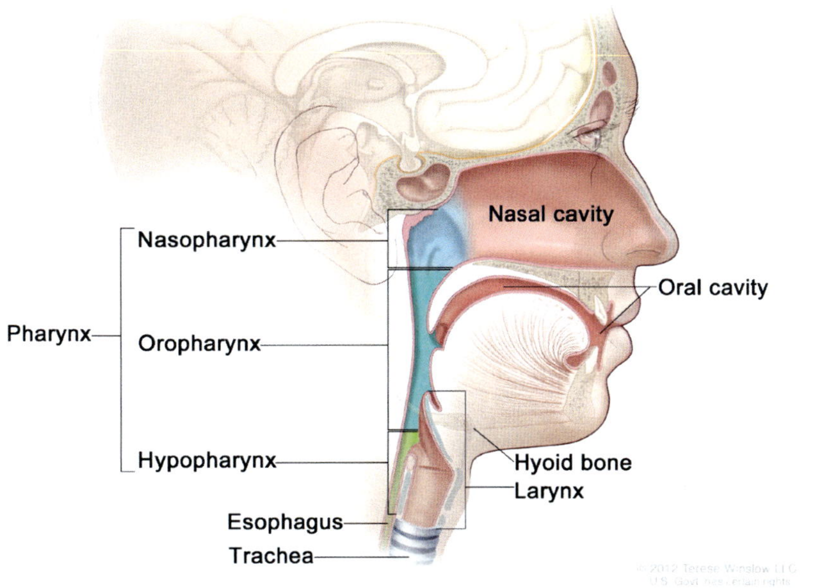

TNM scores

The tumor, node, metastasis (TNM) system is used to stage throat cancer. In this system, the letters T, N, and M describe different areas of cancer growth. Based on imaging and pathology results, a score or number is assigned to each letter. The higher the number, the larger the tumor or the more the cancer has spread. These scores will be combined to assign the cancer a stage. A TNM example might look like this: T1N0M0 or T1, N0, M0.

- **T (tumor) –** Size and extent of the main (primary) tumor
- **N (node) –** If cancer has spread to nearby (regional) lymph nodes
- **M (metastasis) –** If cancer has spread to distant parts of the body or metastasized

Numbered stages

Numbered stages are based on TNM scores. Stages range from stage 0 to stage 4, with 4 being the most advanced. They might be written as stage 0, stage I, stage II, stage III, and stage IV.

Other terms might be used instead of numbered cancer stages.

- **Resectable** – Tumor can be removed completely with surgery.
- **Unresectable** – Tumor cannot be removed completely with surgery. The tumor might involve nearby veins and arteries or other structures making it unsafe to remove.
- **Locoregional or locally advanced** – This refers to a tumor that has spread to tissue, organs, or lymph nodes in the head and neck.
- **Moderately or very advanced disease** – This includes cancer that has spread to parts of the neck such as the base of the skull, larynx, oropharynx, bones and muscles behind the nasal cavity, jaw, and roof of the mouth. It might include cancer in the carotid artery.
- **Metastatic** – This is cancer that has spread to other parts of the body, including lung and distant lymph nodes. This might be referred to as very advanced disease. Not all stage 4 cancers have spread through the blood and are metastatic.

NPC stages

Nasopharyngeal carcinoma (NPC) or cancer starts in the nasopharynx. The following TNM staging information is used for squamous cell carcinoma of the nasopharynx. **See Guide 2**.

T = Tumor

A tumor can grow into nearby structures. Head and neck tumors are measured in centimeters (cm). A baseball is 7 cm, a golf ball is 4 cm, and a pea is 1 cm.

- **T0** – No tumor is found, but neck lymph nodes test positive for Epstein-Barr virus.
- **Tis** – This is carcinoma in situ, meaning that cancerous cells are found only in the squamous cell layer.
- **T1** – Tumor is confined to the nasopharynx or has grown into the oropharynx and/or nasal cavity, but not into the parapharyngeal space. The parapharyngeal space is a triangular area near the pharynx (throat), between the base of the skull and the hyoid bone (the bone under the tongue). It is in the deep tissues of the neck and contains mostly fat, as well as blood vessels (including the carotid artery and jugular vein), nerves, lymph nodes, and parts of the salivary (spit) gland.
- **T2** – Tumor has grown into parapharyngeal space, and/or nearby soft tissue (muscles such as the medial pterygoid, lateral pterygoid, and prevertebral muscles)
- **T3** – Tumor has grown into bony structures at the skull (cranial) base, neck (cervical) vertebra, pterygoid (jaw) structures, and/or paranasal sinuses. The base of the skull is between the bottom of your brain and the structures of your face.
- **T4** – Tumor has grown inside the skull, cranial nerves, hypopharynx, eye (orbit) bones, and/or parotid (spit) gland, and/or grown into the area beyond the lateral pterygoid (jaw) muscle.

Guide 2
Nasopharyngeal cancer stages

Stage 0	• Tis, N0, M0
Stage 1	• T1, N0, M0
Stage 2	• T0 or T1, N1, M0 • T2, N0 or N1, M0
Stage 3	• T0 or T1 or T2, N2, M0 • T3, N0 or N1 or N2, M0
Stage 4A	• T4, N0 or N1 or N2, M0 • Any T, N3, M0
Stage 4B	• Any T, Any N, M1

N = Regional lymph node

There are hundreds of lymph nodes throughout your body. They work as filters to help fight infection and remove harmful things from your body. The head and neck contain a network of more than 300 nodes. They are bound together with muscles nerves, and blood and lymph vessels. Most head and neck tumors spread to neck lymph nodes. Regional lymph nodes are found near the tumor. Cancer found in a regional lymph node is a lymph node metastasis. This is different than a distant metastasis, which is found far from the main tumor in the neck.

- **N0 –** No regional lymph node metastasis is found.
- **N1 –** Metastasis of 6 cm or smaller is found inside 1 lymph node.
- **N2 –** Metastasis of 6 cm or smaller is found inside 1 or more lymph nodes on both sides of the neck, above the cricoid. The cricoid is the ring-shaped cartilage of the larynx.
- **N3 –** Metastasis of larger than 6 cm is found inside 1 or more lymph nodes, or an involved lymph node (of any size) is found below the cricoid.

Lymph nodes in the head and neck

There are over 300 lymph nodes in the head and neck. Most tumors spread to nearby lymph nodes.

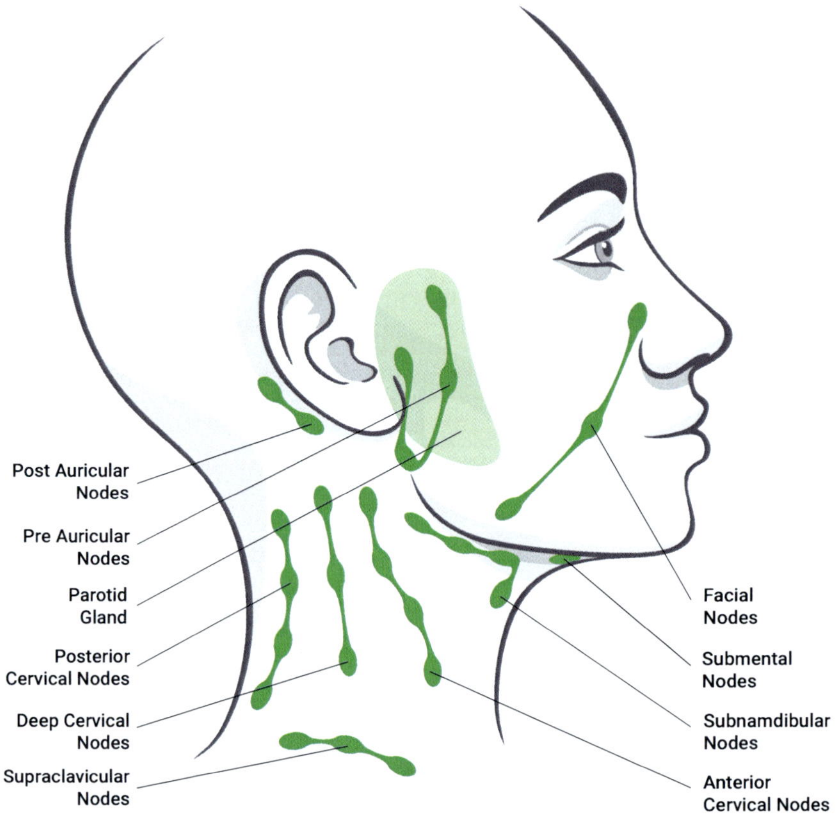

M = Metastasis

Cancer that has spread to distant parts of the body through the bloodstream is shown as M1. The most common sites for metastasis are the lymph nodes outside the head and neck, lungs, or bones.

Key points

- A cancer stage helps to predict the likely course your cancer will take, called a prognosis. It describes the size and location of the tumor and if cancer has spread to lymph nodes, organs, or other parts of the body.
- Staging is only one part of treatment decision-making.
- The head and neck contain a network of more than 300 lymph nodes. They are connected by lymph channels, which drain all areas of the head and neck.
- Most head and neck tumors spread to neck (cervical) lymph nodes.
- Not all stage 4 nasopharyngeal cancers have distant metastases.

Head and neck tumors are measured in centimeters: A baseball is 7 cm, a golf ball is 4 cm, and a pea is 1 cm.

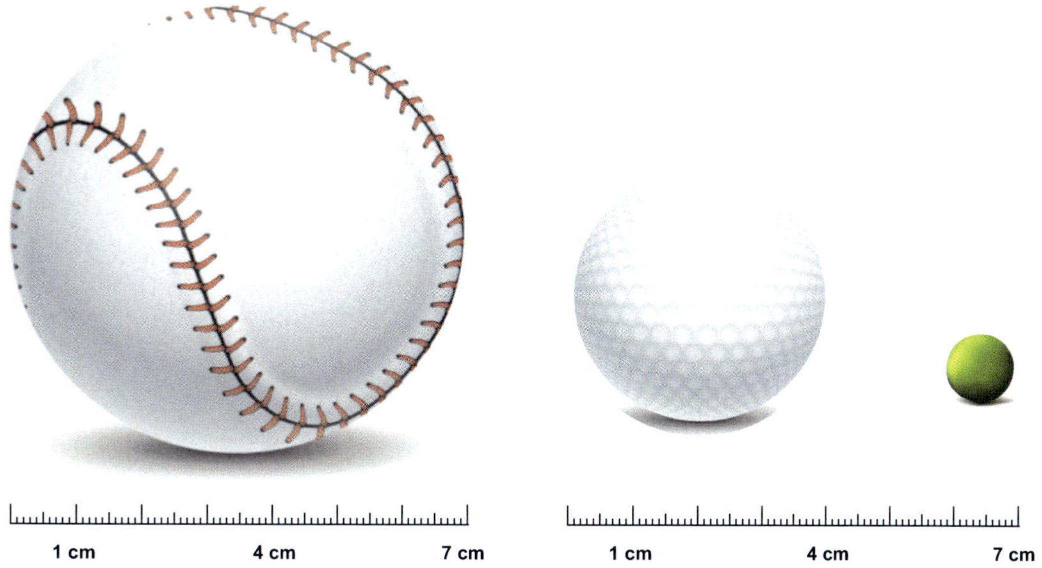

4
Treating nasopharyngeal cancer

Nasopharyngeal cancer is usually treated with a combination of radiation therapy and systemic therapy called chemoradiation. This chapter describes an overview of treatment options and what to expect. Together, you and your care team will choose a treatment plan that is best for you.

Care team

Those with head and cancer should seek treatment at experienced cancer centers.

Treating cancer takes a team approach. Treatment decisions should involve a multidisciplinary team (MDT). An MDT is a team of health care and psychosocial care professionals from different professional backgrounds who have knowledge (expertise) and experience in your type of cancer. This team is united in the planning and implementation of your treatment. Ask who will coordinate your care.

Some members of your care team will be with you throughout cancer treatment, while others will only be there for parts of it. Get to know your care team and help them get to know you.

Depending on your diagnosis, your team might include the following specialists:

- **An otolaryngologist** is an expert in the ear, nose, and throat (ENT).
- **Oncologists** specialize in diagnosing and treating cancer. Types of oncologists include medical, radiation, and surgical oncologists.
- **Oncology nurses** provide your hands-on care, like giving systemic therapy, managing your care, answering questions, and helping you cope with side effects.
- **Oncology pharmacists** are experts in knowing how to use medicines to treat cancer and to manage symptoms and side effects.
- **Palliative care specialists** concentrate on preventing and alleviating suffering and improving quality of life.
- **Radiation therapists** provide your hands-on delivery of radiotherapy treatments.
- **Nutritionists and dietitians** can provide guidance on what foods are most suitable for your condition.
- **An occupational therapist** helps people with the tasks of daily living.
- **A physical therapist** helps people move with greater comfort and ease.
- **A certified lymphedema therapist** gives a type of massage called manual lymph drainage.

- **Speech-language and swallowing therapists** help people who have trouble speaking or swallowing.
- **Psychologists and psychiatrists** are mental health experts who can help manage issues such as depression, anxiety, or other mental health conditions that can affect how you think and feel.
- **Social workers** help people solve and cope with problems in their everyday lives. Clinical social workers also diagnose and treat mental, behavioral, and emotional issues. The anxiety a person feels when diagnosed with cancer might be managed by a social worker in some cancer centers. They, or other designated professionals, can help navigate the complexities of financial and insurance stresses.
- **Spiritual care specialists** identify and support those with spiritual distress or unmet spiritual needs.
- **Smoking cessation specialists** can provide medication and counseling for those who would like to stop using tobacco or nicotine products.
- **A research team** helps to collect research data and coordinate care if you are in a clinical trial. Clinical trials help bring new therapies to patients and advance the treatment for everyone. Consider asking your care team about access to clinical trials.

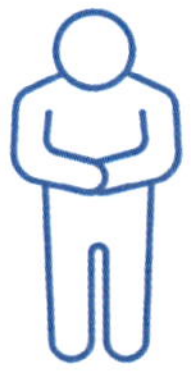

You know your body better than anyone

Help your care team understand:

- ✓ How you feel
- ✓ What you need
- ✓ What is working and what is not

Keep a list of names and contact information for each member of your team. This will make it easier for you and anyone involved in your care to know whom to contact with questions or concerns.

Get to know your care team and help them get to know you.

Radiation therapy

Radiation therapy (RT) uses high-energy radiation from x-rays, photons, electrons, and other sources to kill cancer cells and shrink tumors. RT may be used as main treatment to cure cancer (curative treatment), or as supportive care or palliative care to help ease pain or discomfort caused by advanced cancer. Most types of radiation include short treatment sessions that are given once daily over a few days to weeks. RT treatment can cause a narrowing (stenosis) of the carotid artery, and an RT dose to the carotid artery can increase your risk for stroke. Ask your care team which radiation option(s) are best for your situation, if RT will be combined with chemotherapy, and what side effects to expect.

Panoramic dental x-ray is part of a pre-radiation therapy dental evaluation. It is needed to check the health of your jaw and teeth to see if you need any dental work before starting RT. It is important to tell your dentist about your head and neck cancer and to have regular dental cleanings and checkups.

EBRT

External beam radiation therapy (EBRT) uses a machine outside the body to aim radiation at the tumor(s) or areas of the body.

Common types of EBRT that may be used to treat your cancer include the following:

- **Three-dimensional conformal radiation therapy (3D-CRT)** uses computer software and CT images to aim beams that match the shape of the tumor.
- **Intensity-modulated radiation therapy (IMRT)** uses small beams of different strengths to match the shape of the tumor. This limits the amount of radiation to normal tissue. IMRT is most commonly used to treat NPC.
- **Stereotactic body radiation therapy (SBRT)** uses high-energy proton or photon beams to kill or ablate the tumor. SBRT is very precise, which reduces the chance of damage to nearby tissues.
- **Proton beam therapy (PBT)** uses proton beams to kill or ablate the tumor. It is used as a second radiation option after another type of radiation was used before.

Systemic therapy

Systemic therapy works throughout the body. Types include chemotherapy, targeted therapy, and immunotherapy. Systemic therapy might be used alone or with other therapies such as radiation therapy. Goals of systemic therapy may be curative or palliative and should be discussed before starting treatment. The choice of systemic therapy will be based on your individual needs. Your wishes about treatment are important. Make your wishes known.

For systemic therapy examples, **see Guide 3.**

Chemotherapy

Chemotherapy kills fast-dividing cells throughout the body, including cancer cells and some normal cells. Sometimes, chemotherapies are combined together, or are combined with a checkpoint inhibitor therapy or targeted therapy. This is called multiagent chemotherapy. Chemotherapy might be followed by radiation therapy or chemoradiation.

Chemoradiation

Treatment that combines chemotherapy with radiation therapy is called chemoradiation. Chemotherapy may improve how well radiation works; that is why they are sometimes used together. For locally advanced disease, cisplatin is often the preferred chemotherapy drug given with radiation therapy (RT). Chemoradiation is often used to cure your cancer. Chemoradiation may also be used to control symptoms caused by a tumor even if a cure is not possible.

Guide 3
Systemic therapy examples

Chemotherapy examples	• Capecitabine (Xeloda) • Carboplatin • Cisplatin • Docetaxel (Taxotere)	• 5-fluorouracil (5-FU) • Gemcitabine • Methotrexate • Paclitaxel (Taxol)
Targeted therapy example	• Cetuximab (Erbitux)	
Immunotherapy examples	• Nivolumab (Opdivo) • Pembrolizumab (Keytruda) • Toripalimab-tpzi (Loqtorzi)	

Targeted therapy

Targeted therapy focuses on specific or unique features of cancer cells. Targeted therapies seek out how cancer cells grow, divide, and move in the body. These drugs stop or inhibit the action of molecules that help cancer cells grow and/or survive. If your tumor has certain mutations, targeted therapy might be used.

Immunotherapy

Immunotherapy is a type of systemic treatment that tries to reactivate the immune system against tumor cells. Immunotherapy can be given alone or with other types of treatment. If your tumor has a high number of mutations, immunotherapy might be given.

For more information, see NCCN Guidelines for Patients: Immunotherapy Side Effects, available at NCCN.org/patientguidelines and on the NCCN Patient Guides for Cancer app.

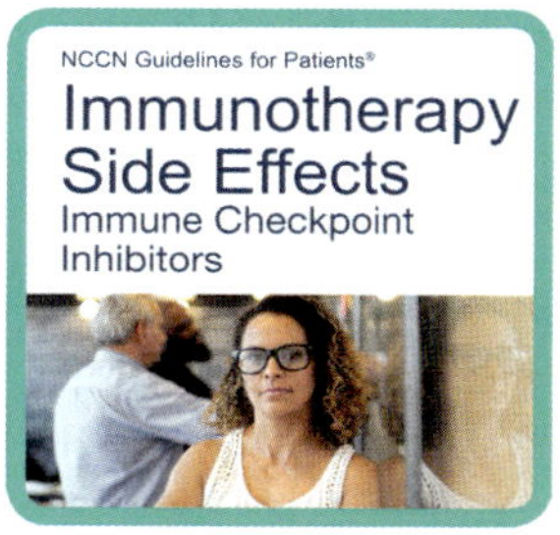

Standard of care is the best-known way to treat a particular disease based on past clinical trials. There may be more than one treatment regimen that is considered standard of care. Ask your care team what treatment options are available and if a clinical trial might be right for you.

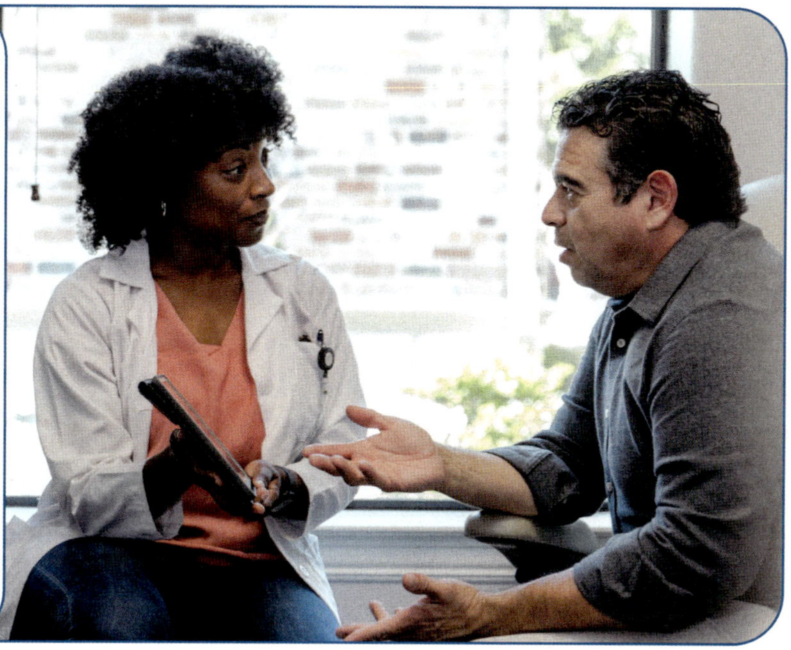

Clinical trials

A clinical trial is a type of medical research study. After being developed and tested in a laboratory, potential new ways of treating cancer need to be studied in people. If found to be safe and effective in a clinical trial, a drug, device, or treatment approach may be approved by the U.S. Food and Drug Administration (FDA).

Everyone with cancer should carefully consider all of the treatment options available for their cancer type, including standard treatments and clinical trials. Talk to your doctor about whether a clinical trial may make sense for you.

Phases

Most cancer clinical trials focus on treatment. Treatment trials are done in phases.

- **Phase I trials** study the dose, safety, and side effects of an investigational drug or treatment approach. They also look for early signs that the drug or approach is helpful.
- **Phase II trials** study how well the drug or approach works against a specific type of cancer.
- **Phase III trials** test the drug or approach against a standard treatment. If the results are good, it may be approved by the FDA.
- **Phase IV trials** study the long-term safety and benefit of an FDA-approved treatment.

Radiation therapy

External beam radiation therapy (EBRT) uses a machine outside the body to aim radiation at the tumor(s) or areas of the body.

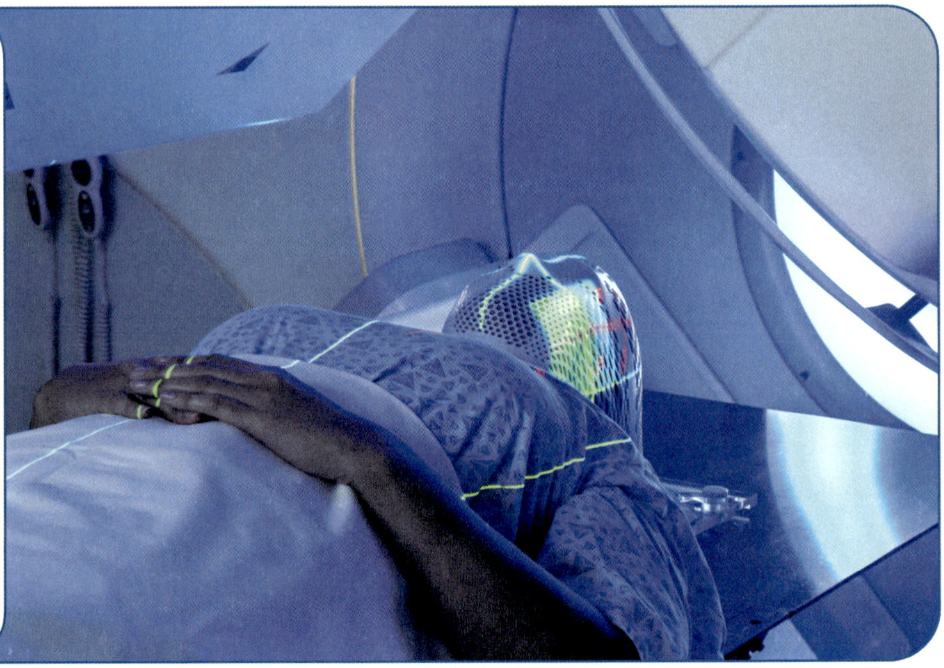

Who can enroll?

Every clinical trial has rules for joining, called eligibility criteria. The rules may be about age, cancer type and stage, treatment history, lab tests, or general health. These requirements ensure that participants are alike in specific ways and that the trial is as safe as possible for the participants.

Informed consent

Clinical trials are managed by a group of experts called a research team. The research team will review the study with you in detail, including its purpose and the risks and benefits of joining. All of this information is also provided in an informed consent form. Read the form carefully and ask questions before signing it. Take time to discuss with family, friends, or others whom you trust. Keep in mind that you can leave and seek treatment outside of the clinical trial at any time.

Start the conversation

Don't wait for your doctor to bring up clinical trials. Start the conversation and learn about all of your treatment options. If you find a study that you may be eligible for, ask your treatment team if you meet the requirements. If you have already started standard treatment you may not be eligible for certain clinical trials. Try not to be discouraged if you cannot join. New clinical trials are always becoming available.

Frequently asked questions

There are many myths and misconceptions surrounding clinical trials. The possible benefits and risks are not well understood by many with cancer.

Will I get a placebo?

Placebos (inactive versions of real medicines) are almost never used alone in cancer clinical trials. It is common to receive either a placebo with a standard treatment, or a new drug with a standard treatment. You will be informed, verbally and in writing, if a placebo is part of a clinical trial before you enroll.

Do I have to pay to be in a clinical trial?

It depends on the study, your health insurance, and the state in which you live. In general, procedures, drugs, or tests that are considered standard of care will be billed to you or your insurance, whereas those considered research are covered by the trial sponsor. Your treatment team and the research team can help determine if you are responsible for any costs.

Supportive care

Supportive care will be specific to your needs. Supportive care is health care given to prevent, reduce, and relieve suffering, and to improve quality of life. Supportive care might include pain relief, palliative care, emotional or spiritual support, financial aid, or family counseling. Tell your care team how you are feeling and about any side effects so they can be managed. Supportive care, best supportive care, and palliative care often mean the same thing.

It is very important to take care of yourself by eating well, drinking plenty of fluids, exercising, and doing things that make you feel energized. Strength is needed to sustain you during treatment.

Side effects

All cancer treatments can cause unwanted health issues called side effects. Side effects depend on many factors. These factors include the drug type and dose, length of treatment, and the person. Some side effects may be harmful to your health. Others may just be unpleasant. Treatment can cause several side effects. Some are very serious.

Ask for a complete list of side effects of your treatments. Also, tell your treatment team about any new or worsening symptoms. There may be ways to help you feel better. There are also ways to prevent some side effects. You will be monitored closely for side effects.

It is important to tell your care team about all of your side effects so they can be managed.

Late effects

Late effects are side effects that occur months or years after a disease is diagnosed or after treatment has ended. Late effects may be caused by cancer or cancer treatment. They may include physical, mental, and social problems, and second cancers. The sooner late effects are treated the better. Ask your care team about what late effects could occur. This will help you know what to look for.

Survivorship

A person is a cancer survivor from the time of diagnosis until the end of life. When treatment leads to remission (or no evidence of disease), you will need follow-up or survivorship care for late effects. During survivorship care you will still have a care team, but it will look different. Seek out peer support groups, whether online or in person.

Side effects

Cranial neuropathies

Cranial neuropathies are a common symptom of nasopharyngeal cancer. Cranial neuropathy affects the nerves in the head and neck and might cause pain; dizziness (vertigo); weakness, numbness, or tingling in the face; or changes in vision, hearing, taste, and smell. These changes can affect speech, swallowing, and hearing, making it difficult to communicate. This might cause distress and impact your ability to function and complete certain tasks at home and at work. Your treatment may not completely reverse these symptoms. Treatment may also worsen or cause new cranial neuropathies if your cancer is located close to a sensitive nerve or brain structures. Ask your doctor about these risks, and what can be done to minimize them. You can also ask to see an occupational therapist or speech-language pathologist (SLP), who might be able to help your recovery from these symptoms.

Difficulty eating, swallowing, or speaking

Because of the location of nasopharyngeal cancer, difficulty eating, swallowing, or speaking are common side effects of treatment. Difficulty swallowing (dysphagia) or painful swallowing (odynophagia) can be caused by treatment and might be long term (chronic). Speech-language pathologists (SLPs) can help people who have trouble swallowing or speaking.

Supportive care resources

More information on supportive care is available at: NCCN.org/patientguidelines and on the NCCN Patient Guides for Cancer app.

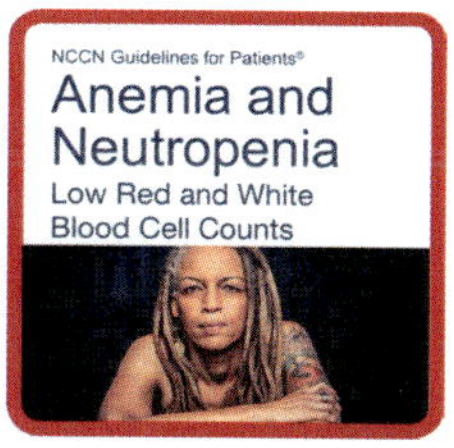

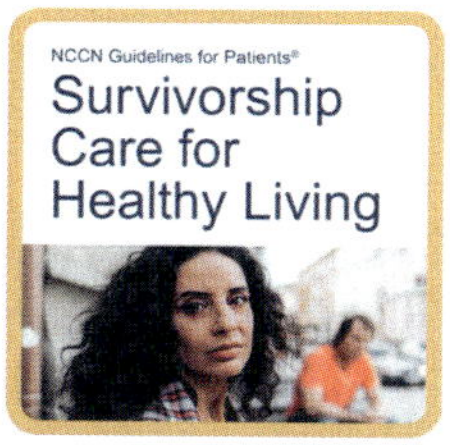

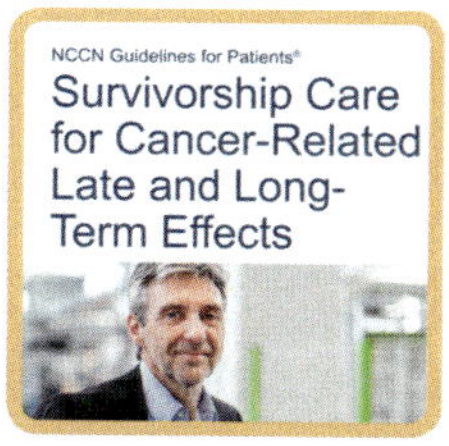

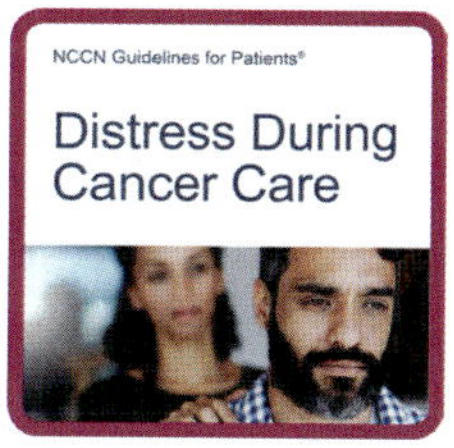

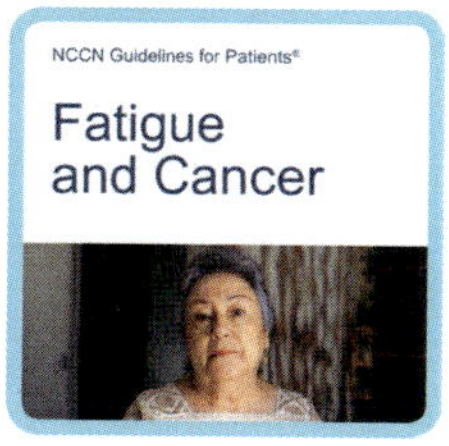

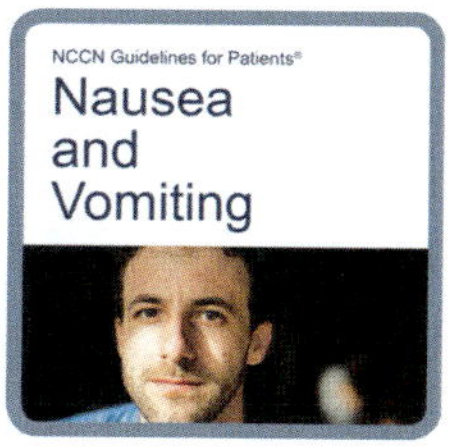

Difficulty with smell, nose bleeds, and congestion

Your sense of smell might be affected by the cancer or its treatment. The lining of your nasal cavity and sinuses might become inflamed or irritated causing your nose to feel stuffed-up or congested. Your nose might bleed. You might have headaches. Your care team might recommend using a humidifier or other ways to help with sinus or nasal irritation.

Distress

Depression, anxiety, and sleeping issues are common and are a normal part of cancer diagnosis. Talk to your care team and with those whom you feel most comfortable about how you are feeling. There are services, people, and medicines that can help you. Support and counseling services are available.

Dry mouth

Xerostomia is the medical term for dry mouth. Treatment to the head or neck can affect your salivary glands. This means you may not make as much spit (saliva) as before and so your mouth may become dry. It is a very common side effect and might be long term (chronic). Drinking plenty of water and avoiding beverages with caffeine, alcohol, or sugar can help. Special mouth rinses are available. Continue to see your dentist regularly.

Fatigue

Fatigue is extreme tiredness and inability to function due to lack of energy. Fatigue may be caused by cancer or it may be a side effect of treatment. Let your care team know how you are feeling and if fatigue is getting in the way of doing the things you enjoy. Eating a balanced diet, exercise, yoga, acupuncture, and massage therapy can help. You might be referred to a nutritionist or dietitian to help with fatigue.

Loss of appetite

Sometimes side effects from cancer or its treatment, and the stress of having cancer might cause you to feel not hungry or sick to your stomach (nauseated). You might have a sore mouth or difficulty swallowing. Healthy eating is important during treatment. It includes eating a balanced diet, eating the right amount of food, and drinking enough fluids. A registered dietitian who is an expert in nutrition and food can help. Weight loss is common in those with head and neck cancer. You might be asked to see a nutrition expert before starting treatment to help prevent severe weight loss.

Low blood cell counts

Some cancer treatments can cause low blood cell counts.

- **Anemia** is a condition where your body does not have enough healthy blood cells, resulting in less oxygen being carried to your cells. You might tire easily if you are anemic.
- **Neutropenia** is a decrease in neutrophils, a type of white blood cell. This puts you at risk for infection.
- **Thrombocytopenia** is a condition where there are not enough platelets found in the blood. This puts you at risk for bleeding.

Lymphedema

Lymphedema is a condition in which lymph fluid builds up in tissues and causes swelling. It may be caused when part of the lymph system is damaged or blocked, such as during surgery to remove lymph nodes, or by radiation therapy. Cancers that block lymph vessels can also cause lymphedema. Swelling usually develops slowly over time. It may develop during treatment, or it may start years after treatment. If you have lymphedema, you may be referred to an expert in lymphedema management. The swelling may be reduced by exercise, massage, compression devices, and other means.

Nausea and vomiting

Nausea and vomiting are common side effects of treatment. You will be given medicine to prevent nausea and vomiting.

Neurocognitive or neuropsychological effects

Some treatments can damage the nervous system (neurotoxicity) causing problems with concentration, memory, and thinking.

Neuropathy

Neuropathy is a nerve problem that causes pain, numbness, tingling, swelling, or muscle weakness in different parts of the body. It usually begins in the hands or feet and gets worse over time. Neuropathy may be caused by cancer or cancer treatment. Most of the time, neuropathy goes away after treatment.

Organ issues

Treatment might cause your kidneys to not work as well as they should.

Pain

Tell your care team about any pain or discomfort. You might meet with a palliative care specialist or with a pain specialist to manage pain. Some people may benefit from palliative radiation therapy to help relieve pain. During this treatment, a radiation beam is focused on the tumor or metastasis.

Quality of life

Cancer and its treatment can affect your overall well-being or quality of life (QOL). Head and neck tumors often impact a person's ability to function such as chew, swallow, speak, and breathe. They can also impact taste, smell, hearing, how your voice sounds, or how you look. It is very important that you are well-prepared and understand how radiation therapy might cause changes to these functions and your appearance.

For more information on quality of life, see NCCN Guidelines for Patients: Palliative Care at NCCN.org/patientguidelines and on the NCCN Patient Guides for Cancer app.

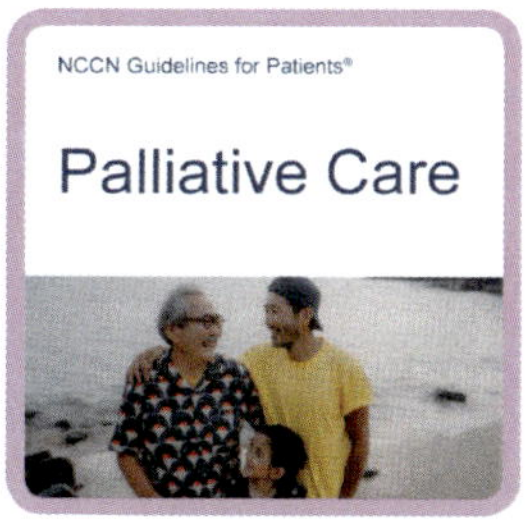

Radiation dermatitis

Radiation dermatitis or radiation burn is a common side effect of radiation therapy. It can cause the skin to change color or cause dry and itchy skin, pain, peeling, blistering, or swelling. Your health care provider can help you find the best treatment for radiation burn.

Stiff neck

Cancer or its treatment can cause a stiff neck and shoulders and long-term (chronic) neck pain. The stress of having cancer can also cause tightness in the neck, shoulders, jaw, and head. Movement such as tai chi, walking, or stretching, and massage might help a stiff neck and shoulders to feel better. Speak to your care team about how to manage chronic neck pain.

Key points

- Systemic therapy works throughout the body. It includes chemotherapy, targeted therapy, and immunotherapy.
- Targeted therapy can block the ways cancer cells grow, divide, and move in the body.
- Immunotherapy uses your body's natural defenses to find and destroy cancer cells.
- Radiation therapy (RT) uses high-energy radiation from x-rays, gamma rays, protons, photons, and other sources to kill cancer cells and shrink tumors.
- Treatment that combines chemotherapy with radiation therapy is called chemoradiation.
- A clinical trial is a type of research that studies a treatment to see how safe it is and how well it works.
- Supportive care is health care that relieves symptoms caused by cancer or its treatment and improves quality of life. Supportive care is always given.
- All cancer treatments can cause unwanted health issues called side effects. It is important for you to tell your care team about all your side effects so they can be managed.
- Eating a balanced diet, drinking enough fluids, exercise, yoga, and massage therapy can help manage side effects.
- Pain may be treated with medication, or radiation with or without systemic therapy. Keeping a pain diary might help you manage pain.

Keep a pain diary

A pain diary is a written record that helps you keep track of when you have pain, how bad it is, what causes it, and what makes it better or worse. Use a pain diary to discuss your pain with your care team. You might be referred to a specialist for pain management.

Include in your pain diary:

- ✓ The time and dose of all medicines
- ✓ When pain starts and ends or lessens
- ✓ Where you feel pain
- ✓ A description of your pain. Is it throbbing, sharp, tingling, shooting, or burning? Is it constant, or does it come and go?
- ✓ Does the pain change at different times of day? When?
- ✓ Does the pain get worse before or after meals? Does certain food or drink make it better?
- ✓ Does the pain get better or worse with activity? What kind of activity?
- ✓ Does the pain keep you from falling asleep at night? Does pain wake you up in the night?
- ✓ A rating of your pain from 0 (no pain) to 10 (worst pain you have ever felt)
- ✓ Does pain get in the way of you doing the things you enjoy?

5 Non-metastatic disease

Treatment is based on tumor location and if any lymph nodes have cancer. Together, you and your care team will choose a treatment plan that is best for you.

Factors such as your overall health are considered when making treatment decisions. Your preferences about treatment are always important. Talk to your care team and make your wishes known.

Early stage

In early-stage cancer, the tumor might be confined to the nasopharynx, or it might have spread to nearby structures. No cancer is found in lymph nodes or a cancer metastasis of 6 cm or smaller may be found in 1 lymph node only. The tumor might test positive for Epstein-Barr virus (EBV+).

Treatment options include:

- Radiation therapy (RT) to the nasopharynx and possibly neck
- RT to the tumor
- Chemoradiation

Locally advanced

The base of the skull is between the bottom of your brain and the structures of your face. It is common for nasopharyngeal cancer to grow into the skull base or very near to it. In locally advanced cancer, the tumor has spread to nearby structures including the skull base and cancer metastasis is in 1 or more lymph

Nasopharyngeal cancer

Cancer can spread from the nasopharynx into or behind the nasal cavity, nearby lymph nodes, and areas such as the oropharynx, base of the skull, jaw, and roof of the mouth. It can also spread to distant sites such as the lung.

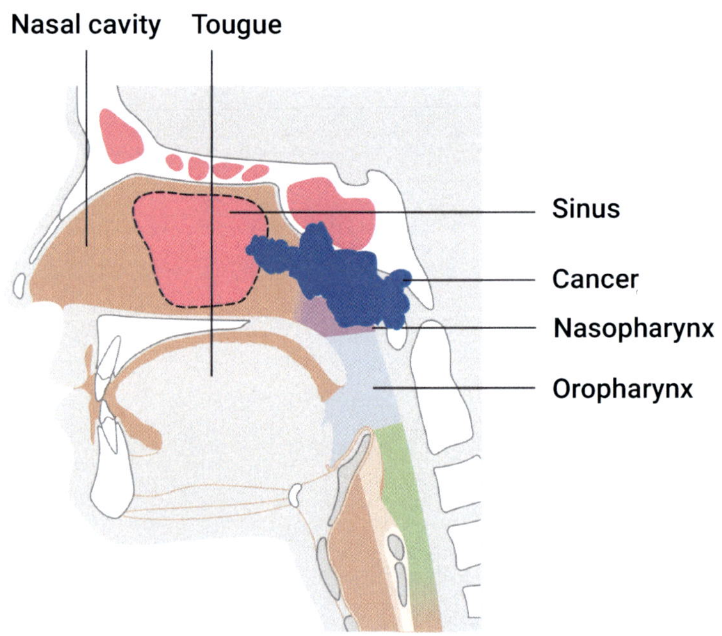

nodes. Cancer has not spread to distant areas in the body.

Treatment options include:

- Clinical trial (preferred)
- Chemotherapy followed by chemoradiation (preferred)
- Chemoradiation followed by chemotherapy
- Chemoradiation alone

Follow-up care

After treatment, you will be monitored for side effects and for any signs of cancer returning (called recurrence). General follow-up care includes regular and frequent doctor visits to check for late effects and signs that cancer has returned. It is important to contact your doctor right away if you notice any changes in your head or neck. For general follow-up care, **see Guide 4.**

Guide 4
Follow-up care

Medical history and physical exam, including complete head and neck exam:

- Year 1, every 1 to 3 months
- Year 2, every 2 to 6 months
- Years 3 through 5, every 4 to 8 months
- Over 5 years, every 12 months

Blood tests to look for hormone levels made by glands in the head and neck

EBV DNA monitoring

Imaging tests as needed

Dental exam for areas exposed to radiation treatment

Supportive care, as needed:

- Speech, hearing, and swallowing evaluation and rehabilitation
- Nutrition evaluation and rehabilitation
- Ongoing screening for depression
- Help to quit smoking; tobacco use and alcohol use counseling
- Lymphedema evaluation and rehabilitation

Information on survivorship care and creation of a survivorship care plan within 1 year of completing treatment

Key points

- In early-stage cancer, the tumor might be found only in the nasopharynx or in nearby structures and cancer may be in 1 lymph node only.
- Treatment options for early-stage cancer are radiation therapy (RT) or chemoradiation.
- In locally advanced cancer, cancer has spread to areas such as the skull and cancer is in 1 or more lymph nodes.
- A clinical trial or chemotherapy followed by chemoradiation is preferred in locally advanced cancer.
- After completing treatment, you will have blood and imaging tests, physical exams, and doctor appointments to monitor for any signs of cancer returning. Contact your doctor right away if you notice any changes in your head or neck.

Warnings about supplements and drug interactions

You might be asked to stop taking or avoid certain herbal supplements when on a systemic therapy. Some supplements can affect the ability of a drug to do its job. This is called a drug interaction.

It is critical to speak with your care team about any supplements you may be taking. Some examples include:

- Turmeric
- Ginkgo biloba
- Green tea extract
- St. John's Wort
- Antioxidants

Certain medicines can also affect the ability of a drug to do its job. Antacids, heart or blood pressure medicine, and antidepressants are just some of the medicines that might interact with a systemic therapy or supportive care medicines given during systemic therapy. Therefore, it is very important to tell your care team about any medicines, vitamins, over-the-counter (OTC) drugs, herbals, or supplements you are taking.

Bring a list with you to every visit.

6
Metastatic disease

This chapter is for cancer that has spread to distant (metastatic) sites. It also includes cancer that remains after treatment (persistent cancer) or cancer that has returned after a disease-free period (recurrence). Together, you and your care team will choose a treatment plan that is best for you.

Factors such as your overall health are considered when making treatment decisions. Your preferences about treatment are always important. Talk to your care team and make your wishes known.

Treatment

Treatment for metastatic disease is based on if there are a few metastases called oligometastases or if the cancer is widespread. Treatment focuses on reducing the number of metastases or amount of cancer, sometimes referred to as cancer burden.

Oligometastatic disease

In oligometastases, a few number of cancer deposits are found outside of the head and neck region.

Treatment options for oligometastases include:

- Chemotherapy followed by radiation therapy (RT) or cisplatin with RT (chemoradiation)
- Cisplatin with RT (chemoradiation)
- Systemic therapy, **see Guide 5**

Widespread disease

Treatment options for widespread metastatic disease include:

- Systemic therapy, **see Guide 5**
- Best supportive care

Supportive care is health care given to prevent, reduce, and relieve suffering, and to improve quality of life. Best supportive care, supportive care, and palliative care often mean the same thing.

Follow-up care

General follow-up care includes regular and frequent doctor visits to check for late effects and signs that cancer has returned. It is important to contact your doctor right away if you notice any changes in your head or neck. For general follow-up care, **see Guide 4**.

Recurrent or persistent disease

Recurrent disease is cancer that has returned after a disease-free period. Persistent disease is cancer that remains after treatment. It might include cancer that has grown or spread during treatment.

Recurrent or persistent disease treatment options are based on:

- If you had radiation therapy before; and
- If the tumor can be removed with surgery (resectable) or cannot be removed with surgery (unresectable).

If surgery is an option

A resectable tumor can be removed with surgery. Surgery is not usually done for nasopharyngeal cancer. This is due to the location of the nasopharynx inside the body.

If surgery is done, it might be followed by radiation therapy (RT), chemoradiation, or a clinical trial. A clinical trial is preferred in some cases. Surgery is not the only option for a resectable tumor. Other options include chemoradiation or systemic therapy followed by RT or chemoradiation.

If surgery is not an option

An unresectable tumor cannot be removed with surgery. Sometimes, an unresectable tumor can become resectable after treatment. Treatment options include chemoradiation, radiation therapy, or systemic therapy.

Guide 5
Systemic therapy options: Recurrent, unresectable, or metastatic disease

Preferred	First-line: • Cisplatin with gemcitabine • Cisplatin with gemcitabine and toripalimab-tpzi • Cisplatin with gemcitabine and pembrolizumab or nivolumab Next-line: • Toripalimab-tpzi (if disease progression on or after platinum-containing therapy)	
Other recommended	First-line combination drugs: • Cisplatin with 5-FU • Cisplatin or carboplatin with docetaxel or paclitaxel • Carboplatin with cetuximab • Gemcitabine with carboplatin Next-line: • Nivolumab or pembrolizumab	First-line single drugs: • Cisplatin • Carboplatin • Paclitaxel • Docetaxel • 5-FU • Methotrexate • Gemcitabine • Capecitabine
Used in some cases	Pembrolizumab (for TMB-H tumors)	

Note: A platinum-based chemotherapy is cisplatin or carboplatin

Key points

- Cancer that has spread to distant areas in the body is called metastatic cancer. Metastatic cancer can be oligometastatic or widespread. In oligometastatic disease, there are a limited number of tumors.
- Recurrent disease is cancer that has returned after a disease-free period. Persistent disease is cancer that remains after treatment. It might include cancer that has grown or spread during treatment.
- Treatment is based on the size and location of the tumor(s), if there is cancer in the lymph nodes, and what treatment you had before. Your overall health and preferences about treatment are also important.
- A resectable tumor can be removed with surgery. An unresectable tumor cannot be removed with surgery. Sometimes an unresectable tumor can become resectable after treatment with chemoradiation, radiation therapy, or systemic therapy.
- After completing treatment, you will have follow-up care to monitor for sides effects and changes in your health. Contact your doctor right away if you notice any changes in your head or neck.

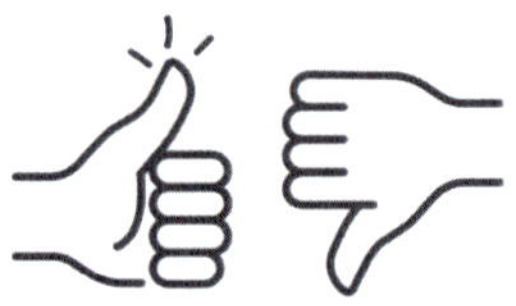

Let us know what you think!

Please take a moment to complete an online survey about the NCCN Guidelines for Patients.

NCCN.org/patients/response

7 Making treatment decisions

It's important to be comfortable with the cancer treatment you choose. This choice starts with having an open and honest conversation with your care team.

It's your choice

In shared decision-making, you and your care team share information, discuss the options, and agree on a treatment plan. It starts with an open and honest conversation between you and your care team.

Treatment decisions are very personal. What is important to you may not be important to someone else. Some things that may play a role in your decision-making:

- What you want and how that might differ from what others want
- Your religious and spiritual beliefs
- Your feelings about certain treatments
- Your feelings about pain or side effects
- Cost of treatment, travel to treatment centers, and time away from school or work
- Quality of life and length of life
- How active you are and the activities that are important to you

Think about what you want from treatment. Discuss openly the risks and benefits of specific treatments and procedures. Weigh options and share concerns with your care team. If you take the time to build a relationship with your care team, it will help you feel supported when considering options and making treatment decisions.

Second opinion

It is normal to want to start treatment as soon as possible. While cancer can't be ignored, there is time to have another doctor review your test results and suggest a treatment plan. This is called getting a second opinion, and it's a normal part of cancer care. Even doctors get second opinions!

Things you can do to prepare:

- Check with your insurance company about its rules on second opinions. There may be out-of-pocket costs to see doctors who are not part of your insurance plan.
- Make plans to have copies of all your records sent to the doctor you will see for your second opinion.

Support groups

Many people diagnosed with cancer find support groups to be helpful. Support groups often include people at different stages of treatment. Some people may be newly diagnosed, while others may be finished with treatment. If your hospital or community doesn't have support groups for people with cancer, check out the websites listed in this book.

Questions to ask

Possible questions to ask your care team are listed on the following pages. Feel free to use these questions or come up with your own. Be clear about your goals for treatment and find out what to expect from treatment.

Questions about testing and diagnosis

1. What tests will I have? How often will they be repeated?
2. Will my insurance pay for this test?
3. How soon will I know the results and who will explain them to me?
4. What will you do to make me comfortable during testing?
5. How will my biopsy be performed? What else might be done at this time?
6. Is my cancer resectable or unresectable? What does this mean?
7. Is the cancer early stage, locally advanced, advanced, or metastatic?
8. Is cancer in any other areas like my lymph nodes or lungs?
9. What does the cancer stage mean in terms of length of survival and quality of life?

Questions about your care team's experience

1. What is your experience treating this cancer? What else do you treat?
2. What is the experience of those on your team?
3. How many people like me (of the same age, gender, race) have you treated?
4. Will you be consulting with experts to discuss my care? Whom will you consult?
5. How many procedures like the one you're suggesting have you done?
6. Is this treatment a major part of your practice?
7. How many of your patients have had complications? What were the complications?
8. How many of these surgeries have you done?
9. Who will manage my day-to-day care?

Questions about options

1. What will happen if I do nothing?
2. How do my age, overall health, and other factors affect the options?
3. Which option is proven to work best for my cancer, age, overall health, and other factors?
4. What are the possible complications and side effects? Are any life-threatening?
5. What can be done to prevent or relieve the side effects of treatment?
6. Am I a candidate for a clinical trial? Can I join a clinical trial at any time?
7. What decisions must be made today?
8. Is there a social worker or someone who can help me decide about treatment?
9. Is there a hospital or treatment center you can recommend for treatment?
10. Can I go to one hospital for surgery and a different center for radiation therapy?

Questions about treatment

1. Which treatment(s) do you recommend and why?
2. Does the order of treatment matter?
3. When will I start treatment?
4. How long will treatment likely take?
5. What should I expect from treatment?
6. What will you do to make me comfortable during treatment?
7. How will treatment affect my ability to taste, smell, chew, breathe, talk, or swallow?
8. Can I work during treatment? When can I go back to work?
9. What are the chances my cancer will return after treatment?
10. I would like a second opinion. Is there someone you can recommend?

Questions about radiation therapy

1. What type of radiation therapy (RT) will I have?
2. What will you target?
3. What is the goal of this RT?
4. How will RT affect my ability to taste, smell, chew, breathe, talk, or swallow?
5. How many treatment sessions will I require? Can you do a shorter course of RT?
6. Do you offer this type of RT here? If not, should I be referred to someone who does?
7. What side effects can I expect from RT?
8. Should I eat or drink before RT?
9. Will I be given medicine to help me relax during RT?
10. What should I wear?

Questions about side effects

1. What are the side effects of this treatment?
2. How are these side effects treated?
3. How long will these side effects last?
4. What side effects should I watch for that could be life-threatening?
5. When should I call my care team?
6. What should I do on weekends and other non-office hours?
7. What emergency department or ER should I go to?
8. Will my treatment team be able to communicate with the ER team?
9. What medicines can I take to prevent or relieve side effects?
10. What can I do to help with pain and other side effects?

Questions about clinical trials

1. What clinical trials are available for my type and stage of cancer?
2. What are the treatments used in the clinical trial?
3. What does the treatment do?
4. Has the treatment been used before? Has it been used for other types of cancer?
5. What are the risks and benefits of this treatment?
6. What side effects should I expect? How will the side effects be controlled?
7. How long will I be in the clinical trial?
8. Will I be able to get other treatments if this doesn't work?
9. How will you know the treatment is working?
10. Will the clinical trial cost me anything? If so, how much?

Questions about resources and support

1. Who can I talk to about help with housing, food, and other basic needs?
2. What help is available for transportation, childcare, and home care?
3. How much will I have to pay for treatment?
4. What help is available to pay for medicines and treatment?
5. What other services are available to me and my caregivers?
6. How can I connect with others and build a support system?
7. How can I find in-person or online support?
8. Who can help me with my concerns about missing work or school?
9. Who can I talk to if I don't feel safe at home, at work, or in my neighborhood?
10. How can I get help to stop smoking or vaping?

Resources

Bag It
bagitcancer.org

Cancer Hope Network
Cancerhopenetwork.org

Head and Neck Cancer Alliance
Headandneck.org

HPV Cancers Alliance
hpvca.org

MedlinePlus
medlineplus.gov/cancers

National Coalition for Cancer Survivorship
canceradvocacy.org

National Cancer Institute (NCI)
cancer.gov/types/head-and-neck

Oral Cancer Foundation
Oralcancerfoundation.org

Support for People with Oral and Head and Neck Cancers
Spohnc.org

THANC Foundation
Thancfoundation.org

Triage Cancer
triagecancer.org

share with us.

Take our survey, and help make the NCCN Guidelines for Patients better for everyone!

NCCN.org/patients/comments

Words to know

biopsy
A procedure that removes fluid or tissue samples to be tested for a disease.

cancer stage
A rating of the growth and spread of cancer.

carcinoma
Cancer that starts in cells that form the lining of organs and structures in the body.

chemotherapy
Drugs that kill cancer cells by damaging or disrupting the making of the genetic code.

clinical stage (c)
Rating the extent of a tumor based on tests before treatment.

clinical trial
Research on a test or treatment to assess its safety or how well it works.

computed tomography (CT)
A test that combines many x-rays to make pictures of the inside of the body.

contrast
A substance put into your body to make clearer pictures during imaging tests.

cricoid
The ring-shaped cartilage of the larynx.

deoxyribonucleic acid (DNA)
A chain of chemicals in cells that contains coded instructions for making and controlling cells.

distant recurrence
Cancer that has come back after treatment and is found in a part of the body far from the first (primary) tumor.

first-line treatment
The first drug or set of drugs given to treat cancer.

gene
Coded instructions in cells for making new cells and controlling how cells behave.

histology
The structure of cells, tissue, and organs as viewed under a microscope.

imaging
A test that makes pictures (images) of the insides of the body.

immune system
The body's natural defense against infection and disease.

immunotherapy
A treatment with drugs that help the body find and destroy cancer cells.

local recurrence
Cancer that has come back after treatment in or near the same place as the first (primary) tumor.

lymph
A clear fluid containing white blood cells.

lymph node
A small group of disease-fighting cells located throughout the body.

lymph vessels
Tubes that carry lymph—a clear fluid containing white blood cells that fight disease and infection—throughout the body and connect lymph nodes to one another.

magnetic resonance imaging (MRI)
A test that uses radio waves and powerful magnets to make pictures of the insides of the body.

medical oncologist
A doctor who's an expert in cancer drugs.

metastasis
The spread of cancer cells from the first tumor to another body part.

mutation
An abnormal change.

nasal cavity
The space inside the nose. The nasal cavity lies above the bone that forms the roof of the mouth and curves down at the back to join the throat. It is divided into 2 sections called nasal passages. Air moves through these passages during breathing. The nasal passages filter and warm the air, and make it moist before it goes into the lungs. They also contain special cells that are involved in the sense of smell.

nasopharynx
The part of the throat that is behind the nose.

oral cavity
Refers to the mouth. It includes the lips, the lining inside the cheeks and lips, the front two thirds of the tongue, the upper and lower gums, the floor of the mouth under the tongue, the bony roof of the mouth, and the small area behind the wisdom teeth.

oropharynx
The middle part of the throat.

palliative care
Treatment for symptoms of a disease. Also sometimes called supportive care.

palliative radiation
Radiation therapy used to relieve symptoms caused by the cancer.

Panorex x-ray
A picture of the inside of the entire mouth, including jaw.

paranasal sinus
One of many small hollow spaces in the bones around the nose. Paranasal sinuses are named after the bones that contain them: frontal (the lower forehead), maxillary (cheekbones), ethmoid (beside the upper nose), and sphenoid (behind the nose). The paranasal sinuses open into the nasal cavity (space inside the nose) and are lined with cells that make mucus to keep the nose from drying out during breathing.

parapharyngeal space
A triangular area near the pharynx (throat), between the base of the skull and the hyoid bone (the bone under the tongue). The parapharyngeal space is in the deep tissues of the neck and contains mostly fat, as well as blood vessels (including the carotid artery and jugular vein), nerves, lymph nodes, and parts of the salivary gland.

pathologic stage (p)
A rating of the extent of cancer based on microscopic review after treatment.

pathologist
A doctor who's an expert in examining tissue and cells to find disease.

positron emission tomography (PET)
A test that uses radioactive material to see the shape and function of body parts.

primary treatment
The main treatment used to rid the body of cancer.

primary tumor
The first mass of cancer cells in the body.

prognosis
The likely course and outcome of a disease based on tests.

radiation oncologist
A doctor who's an expert in radiation treatment.

radiation therapy (RT)
A treatment that uses high-energy rays.

radiologist
A doctor who is an expert in imaging tests.

radiotracer
A substance that releases small amounts of energy (radiation) that is put into the body to make pictures clearer.

recurrence
The return of cancer after a cancer-free period. Also called a relapse.

resectable
Cancer that can be removed with surgery.

side effect
An unhealthy or unpleasant physical or emotional response to treatment

skull base
A group of bones and tissues between the bottom of the brain and the structures of the face.

staging
The process of rating and describing the extent of cancer in the body.

standard of care
The best-known way to treat a particular disease based on past clinical trials. There may be more than one treatment regimen that is considered standard of care.

supportive care
Health care that includes symptom relief but not cancer treatment. Also called palliative care and best supportive care.

targeted therapy
Treatment with drugs that target a specific or unique feature of cancer cells.

throat
A hollow, muscular tube inside the neck that starts behind the nose and ends at the top of the trachea (windpipe) and esophagus (the tube that goes to the stomach).

treatment plan
A written course of action through cancer treatment and beyond.

tumor
An abnormal mass of cells.

ultrasound (US)
A test that uses sound waves to take pictures of the insides of the body.

unresectable
Cancer that can't be completely removed by surgery.

NCCN Contributors

This patient guide is based on the NCCN Clinical Practice Guidelines in Oncology (NCCN Guidelines®) for Head and Neck Cancers Version 1.2024. It was adapted, reviewed, and published with help from the following people:

Dorothy A. Shead, MS
Senior Director
Patient Information Operations

Tanya Fischer, MEd, MSLIS
Senior Medical Writer

Laura Phillips
Graphic Artist

The NCCN Clinical Practice Guidelines in Oncology (NCCN Guidelines®) for Head and Neck Cancers Version 2.2024 were developed by the following NCCN Panel Members:

David G. Pfister, MD
Memorial Sloan Kettering Cancer Center

*Sharon Spencer, MD
O'Neal Comprehensive Cancer Center at UAB

Douglas Adkins, MD
Siteman Cancer Center at Barnes-Jewish Hospital and Washington University School of Medicine

Andrew C. Birkeland, MD
UC Davis Comprehensive Cancer Center

David M. Brizel, MD
Duke Cancer Institute

Paul M. Busse, MD, PhD
Massachusetts General Hospital Cancer Center

Jimmy J. Caudell, MD, PhD
Moffitt Cancer Center

Anthony J. Cmelak, MD
Vanderbilt-Ingram Cancer Center

*A. Dimitrios Colevas, MD
Stanford Cancer Institute

Greg Durm, MD, MS
Indiana University Melvin and Bren Simon Comprehensive Cancer Center

Carole Fakhry, MD, MPH
The Sidney Kimmel Comprehensive Cancer Center at Johns Hopkins

Thomas Galloway, MD
Fox Chase Cancer Center

Jessica L. Geiger, MD
Case Comprehensive Cancer Center/ University Hospitals Seidman Cancer Center and Cleveland Clinic Taussig Cancer Institute

Maura L. Gillison, MD, PhD
The University of Texas MD Anderson Cancer Center

Robert I. Haddad, MD
Dana-Farber/Brigham and Women's Cancer Center

Wesley L. Hicks, Jr., MD
Roswell Park Cancer Institute

Ying J. Hitchcock, MD
Huntsman Cancer Institute at the University of Utah

Antonio Jimeno, MD, PhD
University of Colorado Cancer Center

Debra Leizman, MD
Case Comprehensive Cancer Center/ University Hospitals Seidman Cancer Center and Cleveland Clinic Taussig Cancer Institute

Ellie Maghami, MD
City of Hope National Medical Center

Loren K. Mell, MD
UC San Diego Moores Cancer Center

Bharat B. Mittal, MD
Robert H. Lurie Comprehensive Cancer Center of Northwestern University

Harlan A. Pinto, MD
Stanford Cancer Institute

James W. Rocco, MD, PhD
The Ohio State University Comprehensive Cancer Center - James Cancer Hospital and Solove Research Institute

*Cristina P. Rodriguez, MD
Fred Hutchinson Cancer Center

Panayiotis S. Savvides, MD, PhD
Mayo Clinic Comprehensive Cancer Center

*David Schwartz, MD
The University of Tennessee Health Science Center

Jatin P. Shah, MD, PhD
Memorial Sloan Kettering Cancer Center

David Sher, MD, MPH
UT Southwestern Simmons Comprehensive Cancer Center

Maie St. John, MD, PhD
UCLA Jonsson Comprehensive Cancer Center

He Wang, MD, PhD
Yale Cancer Center Smilow Cancer Hospital

Gregory Weinstein, MD
Abramson Cancer Center at the University of Pennsylvania

Francis Worden, MD
University of Michigan Rogel Cancer Center

Justine Yang Bruce, MD
University of Wisconsin Carbone Cancer Center

Sue S. Yom, MD, PhD
UCSF Helen Diller Family Comprehensive Cancer Center

Weining Zhen, MD
Fred & Pamela Buffett Cancer Center

NCCN

Susan Darlow, PhD
Manager Guidelines Information Standardization

Nicole McMillian, MS
Senior Guidelines Coordinator

Sarah Montgomery, BA
Guidelines Layout Specialist

* Reviewed this patient guide. For disclosures, visit NCCN.org/disclosures.

NCCN Cancer Centers

Abramson Cancer Center
at the University of Pennsylvania
Philadelphia, Pennsylvania
800.789.7366 • pennmedicine.org/cancer

Case Comprehensive Cancer Center/
University Hospitals Seidman Cancer Center and
Cleveland Clinic Taussig Cancer Institute
Cleveland, Ohio
UH Seidman Cancer Center
800.641.2422 • uhhospitals.org/services/cancer-services
CC Taussig Cancer Institute
866.223.8100 • my.clevelandclinic.org/departments/cancer
Case CCC
216.844.8797 • case.edu/cancer

City of Hope National Medical Center
Duarte, California
800.826.4673 • cityofhope.org

Dana-Farber/Brigham and Women's Cancer Center |
Mass General Cancer Center
Boston, Massachusetts
617.732.5500 • youhaveus.org
617.726.5130 • massgeneral.org/cancer-center

Duke Cancer Institute
Durham, North Carolina
888.275.3853 • dukecancerinstitute.org

Fox Chase Cancer Center
Philadelphia, Pennsylvania
888.369.2427 • foxchase.org

Fred & Pamela Buffett Cancer Center
Omaha, Nebraska
402.559.5600 • unmc.edu/cancercenter

Fred Hutchinson Cancer Center
Seattle, Washington
206.667.5000 • fredhutch.org

Huntsman Cancer Institute at the University of Utah
Salt Lake City, Utah
800.824.2073 • healthcare.utah.edu/huntsmancancerinstitute

Indiana University Melvin and Bren Simon
Comprehensive Cancer Center
Indianapolis, Indiana
888.600.4822 • www.cancer.iu.edu

Mayo Clinic Comprehensive Cancer Center
Phoenix/Scottsdale, Arizona
Jacksonville, Florida
Rochester, Minnesota
480.301.8000 • Arizona
904.953.0853 • Florida
507.538.3270 • Minnesota
mayoclinic.org/cancercenter

Memorial Sloan Kettering Cancer Center
New York, New York
800.525.2225 • mskcc.org

Moffitt Cancer Center
Tampa, Florida
888.663.3488 • moffitt.org

O'Neal Comprehensive Cancer Center at UAB
Birmingham, Alabama
800.822.0933 • uab.edu/onealcancercenter

Robert H. Lurie Comprehensive Cancer Center
of Northwestern University
Chicago, Illinois
866.587.4322 • cancer.northwestern.edu

Roswell Park Comprehensive Cancer Center
Buffalo, New York
877.275.7724 • roswellpark.org

Siteman Cancer Center at Barnes-Jewish Hospital
and Washington University School of Medicine
St. Louis, Missouri
800.600.3606 • siteman.wustl.edu

St. Jude Children's Research Hospital/
The University of Tennessee Health Science Center
Memphis, Tennessee
866.278.5833 • stjude.org
901.448.5500 • uthsc.edu

Stanford Cancer Institute
Stanford, California
877.668.7535 • cancer.stanford.edu

The Ohio State University Comprehensive Cancer Center -
James Cancer Hospital and Solove Research Institute
Columbus, Ohio
800.293.5066 • cancer.osu.edu

The Sidney Kimmel Comprehensive
Cancer Center at Johns Hopkins
Baltimore, Maryland
410.955.8964
www.hopkinskimmelcancercenter.org

The UChicago Medicine Comprehensive Cancer Center
Chicago, Illinois
773.702.1000 • uchicagomedicine.org/cancer

The University of Texas MD Anderson Cancer Center
Houston, Texas
844.269.5922 • mdanderson.org

UC Davis Comprehensive Cancer Center
Sacramento, California
916.734.5959 • 800.770.9261
health.ucdavis.edu/cancer

UC San Diego Moores Cancer Center
La Jolla, California
858.822.6100 • cancer.ucsd.edu

UCLA Jonsson Comprehensive Cancer Center
Los Angeles, California
310.825.5268 • cancer.ucla.edu

UCSF Helen Diller Family
Comprehensive Cancer Center
San Francisco, California
800.689.8273 • cancer.ucsf.edu

University of Colorado Cancer Center
Aurora, Colorado
720.848.0300 • coloradocancercenter.org

University of Michigan Rogel Cancer Center
Ann Arbor, Michigan
800.865.1125 • rogelcancercenter.org

University of Wisconsin Carbone Cancer Center
Madison, Wisconsin
608.265.1700 • uwhealth.org/cancer

UT Southwestern Simmons
Comprehensive Cancer Center
Dallas, Texas
214.648.3111 • utsouthwestern.edu/simmons

Vanderbilt-Ingram Cancer Center
Nashville, Tennessee
877.936.8422 • vicc.org

Yale Cancer Center/Smilow Cancer Hospital
New Haven, Connecticut
855.4.SMILOW • yalecancercenter.org

Finding a clinical trial

In the United States

NCCN Cancer Centers
NCCN.org/cancercenters

The National Cancer Institute (NCI)
cancer.gov/about-cancer/treatment/clinical-trials/search

Worldwide

The U.S. National Library of Medicine (NLM)
clinicaltrials.gov

Need help finding a clinical trial?

NCI's Cancer Information Service (CIS)
1.800.4.CANCER (1.800.422.6237)
cancer.gov/contact

Notes

Index

Made in the USA
Las Vegas, NV
20 August 2025

26602642R00040